MENTAL HEALTH MASTERY

For Seniors

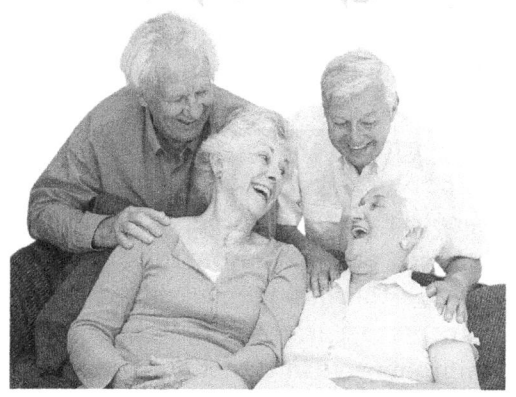

Strategies to Manage Depression
Anxiety and Social Well-being

SIGMUND KING

Copyright © Sigmund King 2024 All rights reserved. Any part of this book must not be copied, stored in a retrieval system, or transmitted in any way or by any means, electronic, mechanical, for photocopying, recording, or otherwise, without the publisher's prior written consent.

Disclaimer Notice: Contained in this book are the property of the Author, Inc. and may not be reproduced, distributed, or transmitted in any form or by any means, electronic, mechanical, photocopying, recording, or otherwise, without prior written permission from the publisher. Every effort has been made to provide accurate, current, trustworthy, and comprehensive information. There are no express or implied warranties of any sort.

For free consultation and assistance on "Mental Health Mastery for Seniors" feel free to contact me with questions or for more information.
SigmundCare@gmail.com

"True wisdom is not found in the absence of struggle, but in the lessons learned and the growth attained through embracing life's challenges"

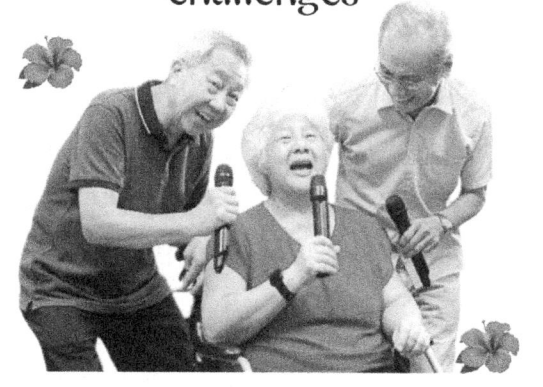

"Strength lies not in avoiding challenges, but in facing them with grace, resilience, and an unwavering belief in one's ability to overcome"

ABOUT THE AUTHOR

Sigmund King, renowned psychologist and advocate for mental health awareness, brings a wealth of expertise and compassion to the pages of "Mental Health Mastery for Seniors." With over three decades of experience in the field, King has dedicated his career to understanding the intricate nuances of the human mind and championing the importance of mental well-being across all ages. As a trusted authority in geriatric psychology, he has worked tirelessly to break down barriers and stigma surrounding mental health issues in the senior community.

King's approach blends empirical research with heartfelt empathy, offering readers not only practical strategies but also a deep understanding of the emotional complexities that seniors may face. His commitment to holistic healing shines through as he guides readers on a transformative journey towards reclaiming joy, purpose, and resilience in their golden years.

Through his insightful writing and compassionate guidance, King empowers seniors to embrace the fullness of life's possibilities, fostering a community of support and encouragement where mental health mastery becomes not just a goal, but a way of life.

TABLE OF CONTENT

- TABLE OF CONTENT 6
- INTRODUCTION 8
- **CHAPTER 1** 11
- **Understanding Mental Health in Later Years** 11
  - Exploring common mental health challenges 14
  - Recognizing signs and symptoms 18
- **CHAPTER 2** 24
- **Coping Strategies and Self-Care** 24
  - Mindfulness and Relaxation Techniques 25
  - Techniques for managing stress and anxiety 29
  - Importance of self-care routines 34
- **CHAPTER 3** 39
- **Maintaining Healthy Relationships** 39
  - Nurturing connections with family and friends 43
  - Dealing with loneliness and social isolation 46
- **CHAPTER 4** 51
- **The Relationship Between Physical and Mental Wellness** 51
  - Exploring the mind-body connection 55
  - Strategies for promoting physical wellness 58
- **CHAPTER 5** 64
- **Overcoming Stigma and Seeking Support** 64
  - Addressing misconceptions about mental health ... 69
  - Encouraging seeking professional help 73
- **CHAPTER 6** 78
- **Adapting to Life Changes** 78

Managing life transitions and retirement.................82
Coping with grief and loss..85
CHAPTER 7.. **89**
Creating a Holistic Mental Health Plan..................... **89**
Building personalised strategies for mental
well-being..92
Resources and tools for ongoing support...............95
CONCLUSION.. **100**

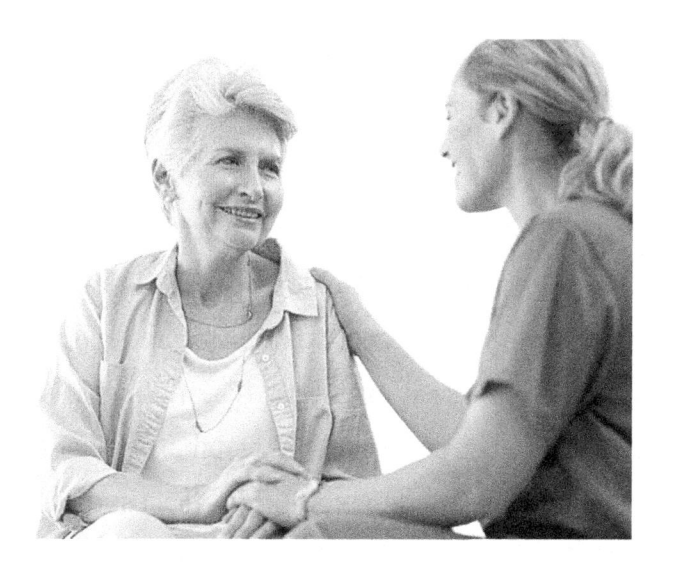

INTRODUCTION

In the quiet corners of ageing, where the sun sets a little softer and the memories dance a little slower, lies a narrative often overlooked—the story of resilience, adaptation, and the unwavering spirit of seniors navigating the complexities of mental health.

Meet Evelyn, an elegant octogenarian whose life once resonated with laughter echoing through bustling streets and the joy of shared moments. Yet, as the years advanced, so did the shadows that crept into her once vibrant world. Loneliness became a frequent visitor, and the weight of past traumas bore heavily on her shoulders, casting a dim haze over her days.

But within Evelyn's tale lies a beacon of hope—a testament to the transformative power of understanding, support, and the unwavering belief in one's ability to heal. As she embarks on a journey of self-discovery and resilience, she uncovers the keys to mental fortitude, unlocking the door to a life of renewed purpose, connection, and inner peace.

In "Thriving Minds: Mental Health Mastery for Seniors," we delve into the heart of Evelyn's narrative, weaving her experiences with actionable insights, empowering strategies, and compassionate guidance tailored specifically for seniors navigating the labyrinth of mental health challenges. Through poignant anecdotes, expert advice, and practical exercises, this book serves as a roadmap to not only surviving but thriving in the golden years, reclaiming joy, and embracing the boundless possibilities that lie ahead.

Join us on a transformative odyssey where age becomes a mere whisper in the symphony of resilience, and the pursuit of mental well-being knows no bounds. Together, let us embark on a journey of discovery, empowerment, and the unyielding pursuit of thriving minds.

CHAPTER 1

Understanding Mental Health in Later Years

Understanding mental health in later years encompasses various aspects. As individuals age, they often encounter unique challenges that can affect their mental well-being. Exploring this topic involves delving into the common mental health issues prevalent among seniors over 50 and recognizing the signs and symptoms associated with these conditions.

One significant aspect is the prevalence of mood disorders such as depression and anxiety. While these conditions can occur at any age, they can manifest differently in older adults due to factors like life changes, health issues, or social isolation. Seniors might mistake symptoms of depression for normal feelings associated with ageing, leading to underreporting and undertreatment. Hence, shedding light on these distinctions is crucial.

Additionally, cognitive health is a vital component. Understanding the difference between normal cognitive changes and potential signs of cognitive decline or dementia is essential. Age-related memory lapses might differ from the concerning memory impairment indicative of cognitive disorders. Educating individuals about these differences empowers them to seek timely intervention if necessary.

Exploring the impact of chronic illnesses on mental health is also imperative. Seniors often grapple with health conditions that can influence their emotional well-being. Chronic pain, for instance, can contribute to feelings of frustration, hopelessness, or anxiety, affecting mental health. Addressing the interplay between physical health and mental well-being helps individuals comprehend the holistic nature of health in later years.

Moreover, the importance of social connections cannot be overstated. Loneliness and social isolation significantly impact mental health among seniors. Understanding the significance of maintaining relationships, engaging in social activities, and seeking support networks can profoundly influence mental well-being.

Lastly, dispelling myths and misconceptions about mental health among seniors is essential. Overcoming stigma associated with seeking mental health support is crucial for fostering an environment where individuals feel comfortable discussing their struggles and seeking appropriate help.

Understanding mental health in later years involves a multifaceted approach. It requires recognizing the nuances of common mental health issues, distinguishing between normal ageing and potential concerns, addressing the impact of physical health, emphasising social connections, and challenging stigmas. By providing comprehensive insights into these aspects, seniors can be better equipped to navigate and prioritise their mental well-being in their later years.

Exploring common mental health challenges

Exploring common mental health challenges faced by seniors over 50 reveals a landscape filled with various intricacies and vulnerabilities. As individuals age, they encounter a multitude of factors that can significantly impact their mental well-being.

Firstly, depression stands out as a prevalent mental health issue among seniors. While sadness is a normal part of life, persistent feelings of sadness, hopelessness, or disinterest in activities once enjoyed could signal depression. Older adults might attribute these symptoms to life changes or health issues, leading to underreporting and undertreatment. Addressing the specific triggers and nuances of late-life depression becomes pivotal in facilitating effective support and interventions.

Anxiety disorders also manifest uniquely in older adults. Seniors may experience excessive worry, fear, or restlessness, often linked to health concerns, financial worries, or the fear of losing independence. Understanding the manifestations of anxiety and its impact on daily life enables tailored strategies for managing and mitigating its effects.

Another prominent challenge is the prevalence of cognitive disorders, including dementia and Alzheimer's disease. Cognitive decline can be distressing and significantly impact an individual's quality of life. Early detection, understanding the warning signs, and distinguishing between normal ageing and more severe cognitive impairments are crucial components in navigating these challenges.

Moreover, the experience of grief and loss becomes more frequent as one ages. Coping with the loss of loved ones, physical abilities, or independence can lead to feelings of isolation, sadness, and even exacerbate existing mental health issues. Providing support and coping mechanisms to navigate these life changes becomes paramount.

Chronic illnesses, prevalent in older age, are intricately linked to mental health challenges. Conditions like arthritis, heart disease, or diabetes not only affect physical health but also contribute to emotional distress. Chronic pain, in particular, can significantly impact mental well-being, leading to feelings of frustration, depression, or anxiety.

Furthermore, social isolation and loneliness emerge as significant mental health challenges among seniors. Changes in social circles due to retirement, loss of friends or family members, or physical limitations can lead to feelings of loneliness. Understanding the importance of maintaining social connections and actively seeking new ones is vital for mitigating the negative impact of isolation on mental health.

In addressing these common mental health challenges, it's imperative to adopt a multifaceted approach. Encouraging open conversations about mental health, normalising seeking help, and providing accessible resources and support networks tailored to the needs of seniors are crucial steps. Implementing community programs, support groups, or educational initiatives targeted at this demographic fosters an environment where individuals feel comfortable discussing their mental health concerns.

Ultimately, navigating mental health challenges among seniors over 50 requires a comprehensive understanding of the diverse issues they face. By acknowledging the multifaceted nature of these challenges and implementing targeted strategies, we can empower older adults to prioritise their mental well-being, thereby enhancing their overall quality of life in their later years.

Recognizing signs and symptoms

Recognizing signs and symptoms of mental health issues among seniors over 50 is crucial in facilitating early intervention and support. As individuals age, they might encounter changes in mental health that differ from those experienced in younger years. Understanding these nuances is key to effectively identifying potential concerns and providing appropriate assistance.

1.Depression

Seniors may exhibit signs of depression that differ from those seen in younger individuals. Persistent feelings of sadness, hopelessness, or lack of interest in previously enjoyable activities are common.

Moreover, physical symptoms such as changes in appetite, sleep disturbances, or unexplained aches and pains might accompany emotional distress. Recognizing these subtler signs is essential for identifying depression in older adults.

2. Anxiety

Anxiety among seniors might manifest as excessive worry about health, finances, or future uncertainties. Physical symptoms like restlessness, trembling, or fatigue might be present alongside persistent anxious thoughts. Understanding the psychological and physical manifestations of anxiety aids in identifying and addressing these concerns in older individuals.

3. Cognitive Changes

Recognizing cognitive changes is crucial. Memory lapses or occasional forgetfulness are normal parts of ageing, but significant changes in memory, language, problem-solving abilities, or disorientation warrant attention. Distinguishing between age-related memory decline and symptoms of cognitive disorders like Alzheimer's disease helps in timely interventions and support.

4. Grief and Loss

Seniors frequently experience loss, whether through the passing of loved ones, retirement, or declining health. Recognizing prolonged feelings of grief, social withdrawal, or persistent sadness after a loss is essential. These signs might indicate a need for additional support to navigate through the grieving process.

5. Chronic Illness Impact

Chronic illnesses prevalent in older age can exacerbate mental health challenges. Recognizing signs of distress or changes in mood associated with chronic conditions like chronic pain, heart disease, or diabetes is important. Physical symptoms affecting mental well-being should not be overlooked.

6. Social Isolation and Loneliness

Observing changes in social behaviour is crucial in identifying loneliness or social isolation. Seniors might withdraw from social activities, exhibit changes in communication patterns, or express feelings of loneliness. Recognizing these signs can prompt interventions aimed at enhancing social connections and reducing isolation.

7. Behavioural Changes

Observing changes in behaviour is significant. Uncharacteristic behaviours such as increased irritability, agitation, withdrawal, or significant changes in routine could signal underlying mental health concerns.

Understanding these signs and symptoms requires a nuanced approach that accounts for the unique experiences of older adults. Education and awareness programs geared towards caregivers, family members, and healthcare professionals can aid in enhancing recognition and response to mental health concerns in seniors.

Moreover, fostering an open dialogue about mental health within communities allows for early identification and destigmatized seeking help. Implementing regular mental health screenings during healthcare check-ups for seniors can also aid in identifying potential issues before they escalate.

Recognizing signs and symptoms of mental health issues among seniors over 50 involves acknowledging the unique manifestations these concerns can have in older adults. By promoting awareness, educating caregivers, and implementing proactive measures, we can facilitate early identification and interventions, ultimately enhancing the mental well-being of this demographic.

CHAPTER 2

Coping Strategies and Self-Care

Coping strategies and self-care play pivotal roles in nurturing the mental well-being of seniors over 50. As individuals age, they encounter various stressors and life changes that necessitate adaptive strategies to maintain their psychological health. Exploring these coping mechanisms and emphasising self-care practices tailored for this demographic is crucial in promoting resilience and enhancing overall mental wellness.

Mindfulness and Relaxation Techniques

Encouraging seniors to practise mindfulness, meditation, or relaxation exercises can significantly alleviate stress and promote emotional balance. Techniques such as deep breathing, progressive muscle relaxation, or guided imagery empower individuals to manage anxiety and reduce the impact of stressors in their daily lives.

1. Physical Activity and Exercise

Engaging in regular physical activity not only benefits physical health but also has profound effects on mental well-being. Encouraging seniors to incorporate exercises suitable for their abilities, such as walking, yoga, or tai chi, can boost mood, reduce anxiety, and enhance overall psychological health.

2. Healthy Lifestyle Choices

Emphasising the importance of nutrition, adequate sleep, and avoiding harmful substances like excessive alcohol or tobacco contributes significantly to mental well-being. Proper nutrition and sufficient rest promote cognitive function and emotional stability in older adults.

3. Cognitive Stimulation

Engaging in mentally stimulating activities, such as puzzles, reading, learning new skills, or participating in educational programs, can preserve cognitive abilities and contribute to a sense of accomplishment and fulfilment.

4. Social Engagement and Support Networks

Encouraging active participation in social activities and fostering connections with friends, family, or community groups is vital. Strengthening social networks reduces feelings of isolation and provides emotional support crucial for maintaining mental health.

5. Establishing Routines and Structure

Creating and maintaining routines can provide a sense of stability and purpose. Structured daily activities, hobbies, or volunteer work contribute to a sense of fulfilment and reduce feelings of aimlessness or boredom.

6. Self-Compassion and Acceptance

Encouraging self-compassion and acceptance of life changes associated with ageing is crucial. Learning to adapt to new circumstances, accepting limitations, and being kind to oneself fosters resilience and emotional well-being.

7. Engagement in Hobbies and Interests

Encouraging seniors to pursue hobbies or interests they enjoy cultivates a sense of purpose and joy. Whether it's gardening, painting, music, or other hobbies, these activities contribute to emotional fulfilment and mental stimulation.

8. Time for Relaxation and Leisure

Emphasising the importance of leisure time and relaxation allows seniors to recharge and reduce stress levels. Engaging in activities that bring joy and relaxation, such as reading, listening to music, or spending time in nature, is crucial for overall well-being.

Tailoring coping strategies and self-care practices to match individual preferences and abilities is essential. Educational programs, community initiatives, or support groups that provide guidance on these strategies can empower seniors to proactively manage their mental health.

Coping strategies and self-care practices are integral components of maintaining mental well-being for seniors over 50. By promoting a holistic approach that encompasses physical, emotional, and social aspects, we empower individuals to navigate life's challenges and enjoy fulfilling and mentally healthy lives in their later years.

Techniques for managing stress and anxiety

Managing stress and anxiety is crucial for maintaining optimal mental health, especially for seniors over 50 who may encounter unique stressors associated with ageing. Implementing effective techniques tailored to this demographic can significantly alleviate these burdens and promote emotional well-being.

1. Deep Breathing Exercises

Encouraging seniors to practise deep breathing exercises can be immensely beneficial. Techniques such as diaphragmatic breathing or guided breathing exercises help in calming the nervous system, reducing stress hormones, and promoting relaxation.

2. Mindfulness and Meditation

Introducing mindfulness practices and meditation techniques can aid in managing stress and anxiety. Mindfulness involves focusing on the present moment, allowing individuals to observe their thoughts and emotions without judgement. This practice cultivates a sense of calm and reduces anxiety.

3. Progressive Muscle Relaxation (PMR)

PMR entails methodically tense and release various bodily muscle groups. This technique helps in releasing physical tension, promoting relaxation, and reducing the physiological effects of stress.

4. Yoga or Tai Chi

Engaging in gentle forms of exercise like yoga or tai chi not only benefits physical health but also promotes mental well-being. These practices incorporate movement, breathing, and meditation, contributing to stress reduction and emotional balance.

5. Journaling and Expressive Writing

Encouraging seniors to maintain a journal or engage in expressive writing allows them to process their thoughts and emotions. Writing about experiences, feelings, or concerns can serve as an outlet for stress and anxiety.

6. Visualization and Guided Imagery

Guided imagery involves imagining calming scenes or situations to reduce stress. Seniors can engage in guided visualisation exercises, picturing tranquil environments or peaceful scenarios to alleviate anxiety and promote relaxation.

7. Engaging in Creative Activities

Encouraging participation in creative activities like painting, drawing, or crafting provides an outlet for self-expression and stress relief. Engaging in these activities can divert attention from stressors and induce relaxation.

8. Setting Boundaries and Prioritising Tasks

Teaching seniors the importance of setting boundaries and managing their commitments can reduce feelings of overwhelm. Helping them prioritise tasks and focus on essential activities alleviates stress associated with feeling overburdened.

9. Limiting Exposure to Stressful Stimuli

Encouraging seniors to limit exposure to stressful stimuli, such as excessive news consumption or negative environments, is crucial. Creating a peaceful and supportive environment aids in managing stress and anxiety levels.

10. Engaging in Relaxation Techniques

Incorporating relaxation techniques such as listening to calming music, taking warm baths, or practising aromatherapy promotes relaxation and reduces stress levels.

Empowering seniors with a variety of techniques enables them to choose those that resonate with their preferences and lifestyles. Providing guidance through community programs, workshops, or educational materials can facilitate the adoption of these stress management techniques.

Employing tailored techniques for managing stress and anxiety among seniors over 50 is vital for their overall well-being. By implementing these strategies, individuals can proactively mitigate the effects of stressors associated with ageing, leading to a more relaxed and fulfilling life.

Importance of self-care routines

Self-care routines hold immense significance in nurturing the overall well-being of seniors over 50. Establishing and maintaining self-care practices tailored to their needs allows individuals to prioritise their physical, mental, and emotional health, fostering a sense of empowerment and resilience.

1.Physical Health Maintenance

Self-care routines encompass various aspects of physical health, including proper nutrition, regular exercise, and adequate sleep. Seniors benefit from maintaining a balanced diet rich in nutrients essential for their age group. Exercise tailored to their abilities aids in maintaining mobility, strength, and overall health. Ensuring sufficient rest contributes to improved energy levels and supports overall physical well-being.

2. Emotional Wellness and Stress Management

Self-care routines play a pivotal role in managing stress and nurturing emotional wellness. Engaging in activities that promote relaxation, such as meditation, deep breathing exercises, or engaging in hobbies, helps in reducing stress levels. Allocating time for leisure and self-reflection allows seniors to tend to their emotional needs and maintain a healthy mindset.

3. Promoting Mental Health

Self-care practices are crucial in supporting mental health. Seniors benefit from engaging in cognitive activities that stimulate their minds, such as puzzles, reading, or learning new skills. Establishing routines and structure in daily activities fosters a sense of purpose and stability, contributing to mental well-being.

4. Preventing Burnout and Compassion Fatigue

Seniors often find themselves in caregiving roles for family members or actively involved in community activities. Self-care routines prevent burnout and compassion fatigue by emphasising the importance of setting boundaries, prioritising personal needs, and seeking support when necessary. Taking breaks and engaging in activities solely for personal enjoyment or relaxation revitalises their spirits.

5. Enhancing Self-Compassion and Esteem

Self-care routines encourage self-compassion and the cultivation of positive self-esteem. Engaging in activities that promote self-acceptance, such as journaling, self-reflection, or affirmations, fosters a positive self-image and self-worth.

6. Preventative Health Measures

Incorporating preventative health measures into self-care routines is essential for seniors. This includes attending regular medical check-ups, following prescribed treatments, and monitoring their health. Self-care routines emphasise the importance of taking proactive steps to maintain health and prevent potential health complications.

7.Promoting Independence and Autonomy

Self-care routines empower seniors to maintain a sense of independence and autonomy in managing their health. By establishing personalised routines, seniors actively participate in their well-being, fostering a sense of control over their lives.

8.Improving Quality of Life

Ultimately, self-care routines significantly contribute to enhancing the overall quality of life for seniors. Prioritising self-care allows them to enjoy their lives, engage in activities they love, and navigate challenges with resilience and confidence.

Encouraging the adoption of self-care routines involves education, support, and the provision of resources tailored to the unique needs and preferences of seniors. Empowering individuals to establish and maintain these practices promotes holistic well-being, enabling them to lead fulfilling lives in their later years.

CHAPTER 3

Maintaining Healthy Relationships

Maintaining healthy relationships is fundamental for the emotional and mental well-being of seniors over 50. Nurturing connections with family, friends, and the community contributes significantly to their overall quality of life and serves as a protective factor against isolation and mental health concerns.

1. Family Bonds

Seniors often derive immense support and companionship from their family members. Maintaining healthy relationships within the family involves regular communication, spending quality time together, and expressing care and appreciation. Strong family bonds provide a sense of belonging and emotional support crucial for seniors' well-being.

2. Friendship and Social Connections

Cultivating friendships and maintaining social connections outside the family circle is equally vital. Seniors benefit from engaging in social activities, clubs, or community groups where they can connect with peers who share similar interests. These connections combat feelings of loneliness and provide opportunities for social engagement and emotional support.

3. Communication and Openness

Effective communication forms the bedrock of healthy relationships. Encouraging open and honest communication among seniors fosters understanding, resolves conflicts, and strengthens connections. Sharing feelings, concerns, and joys with loved ones helps in maintaining strong and supportive relationships.

4. Respecting Boundaries and Autonomy

Respecting each other's boundaries and autonomy is essential in healthy relationships. Seniors should feel empowered to express their preferences and make choices regarding their social interactions and engagements. Respecting their autonomy fosters a sense of dignity and self-worth.

5. Quality Time and Shared Activities

Spending quality time together and engaging in shared activities enhances relationships. Whether it's pursuing hobbies, going for walks, or simply enjoying conversations, these shared experiences create bonds and strengthen connections among seniors and their loved ones.

6. Forging New Connections

Encouraging seniors to forge new connections is important, especially after life transitions like retirement or relocation. Joining clubs, attending community events, or volunteering opportunities provides avenues to meet new people and establish meaningful relationships.

7. Conflict Resolution and Forgiveness

Encouraging seniors to address conflicts and practice forgiveness is crucial. Resolving disagreements and letting go of resentments promotes healthier relationships, reducing stress and improving overall emotional well-being.

8. Support Networks and Resources

Encouraging seniors to access support networks or resources designed for their age group helps in expanding their social connections. Community centres, support groups, or senior-specific activities provide platforms for interaction and support.

Promoting healthy relationships among seniors involves not only nurturing existing connections but also encouraging the development of new ones. Educational programs, workshops, or social activities tailored for seniors facilitate opportunities for social engagement and relationship-building, ultimately contributing to their happiness and well-being.

Nurturing connections with family and friends

Nurturing connections with family and friends holds profound significance for seniors over 50, contributing significantly to their emotional well-being and overall quality of life.

1. Quality Time and Shared Memories
Spending quality time with family and friends creates cherished memories and strengthens bonds. Whether through regular visits, shared meals, or engaging in activities together, these experiences foster a sense of belonging and emotional closeness.

2. Emotional Support and Companionship
Family and friends often serve as pillars of emotional support. Their presence provides

comfort during challenging times, offering a listening ear and a source of encouragement. Seniors feel reassured and valued when they can rely on their loved ones for support.

3.Communication and Connection
Regular communication helps maintain connections. Whether through phone calls, video chats, or in-person visits, staying in touch enables seniors to feel connected and involved in the lives of their family and friends, reducing feelings of loneliness or isolation.

4.Celebrating Milestones and Traditions
Sharing in celebrations, milestones, and traditions strengthens familial and friendship bonds. Participating in holidays, birthdays, and other significant events fosters a sense of togetherness and continuity within relationships.

5.Mutual Assistance and Care

Healthy relationships involve reciprocity. Seniors contribute to their relationships by providing wisdom, support, and care, while also receiving assistance and care from their loved ones when needed. This mutual exchange strengthens connections and deepens trust.

6. Creating Support Networks

Encouraging seniors to create broader support networks within their family and friend circles is beneficial. It allows for a wider range of connections, ensuring a diverse support system that caters to different needs and interests.

7. Adapting to Changing Circumstances

Nurturing connections involves adapting to changing circumstances, such as life transitions or geographical distances. Embracing change and finding new ways to connect, even if it's through technology or occasional visits, maintains the strength of relationships.

8. Fostering connections with family and friends

Requires active participation and investment from both sides. Seniors benefit immensely from these connections, experiencing emotional fulfilment, support, and a sense of belonging within their social circles.

Dealing with loneliness and social isolation

Dealing with loneliness and social isolation among seniors over 50 is crucial for maintaining their mental and emotional well-being. Several strategies can help mitigate these feelings and foster a sense of connection and belonging.

1. Building Social Connections

Encouraging seniors to proactively seek social connections is vital. Engaging in community groups, clubs, or volunteering opportunities creates opportunities for interaction and companionship, reducing feelings of isolation.

2. Utilising Technology for Connection

Embracing technology enables seniors to stay connected with family and friends, especially if distance hinders in-person interactions. Video calls, social media, or online communities provide platforms for communication and engagement.

3. Participating in Group Activities

Involvement in group activities tailored for seniors fosters a sense of belonging. Joining book clubs, fitness classes, or hobby groups not only provides opportunities for social interaction but also shared interests and experiences.

4. Seeking Support Services

Encouraging seniors to access support services or counselling when dealing with loneliness is essential. Support groups or counselling sessions catered to their needs provide a safe space for sharing experiences and receiving emotional support.

5. Fostering Intergenerational Connections
Encouraging interactions with younger generations, such as through mentoring programs or involvement in community initiatives, provides a sense of purpose and connection, reducing feelings of isolation.

6. Pets as Companions
Pets can offer companionship and emotional support. The presence of a pet can alleviate feelings of loneliness and provide comfort and companionship for seniors.

7. Encouraging Hobbies and Activities
Engaging in hobbies or activities that bring joy and fulfilment is crucial. Pursuing interests or learning new skills not only occupies time but also offers opportunities for social engagement and connection.

8.Addressing Mobility and Accessibility

Overcoming barriers to mobility or accessibility issues enables seniors to participate in social activities more easily. Accessible transportation or modifications to living spaces can facilitate social engagement.

By implementing these strategies and fostering an environment that supports social connections, seniors can combat feelings of loneliness and social isolation. Encouraging participation in diverse activities and providing access to various support systems contributes significantly to their overall well-being.

CHAPTER 4

The Relationship Between Physical and Mental Wellness

The intricate relationship between physical health and mental well-being among seniors over 50 is profound, showcasing how one significantly influences the other. Maintaining optimal physical health positively impacts mental wellness, contributing to a better quality of life.

1. Exercise and Mental Health

Engaging in regular physical activity offers numerous mental health benefits. Exercise stimulates the release of endorphins, neurotransmitters that elevate mood and reduce feelings of stress or anxiety. Additionally, physical activity promotes better sleep patterns, contributing to improved mental clarity and emotional stability.

2. Nutrition and Brain Function

Proper nutrition is crucial for maintaining cognitive function and emotional well-being. A balanced diet rich in essential nutrients supports brain health, influencing mood regulation and cognitive abilities. Nutritional deficiencies can contribute to mental health issues such as depression or anxiety.

3. Mind-Body Connection

The mind-body connection is evident in how physical health impacts mental well-being. Chronic health conditions, such as heart disease or diabetes, not only affect the body but also impact mental health. Managing these conditions effectively is vital in preventing associated mental health challenges.

4. Pain Management and Emotional Health

Chronic pain significantly affects mental well-being. Seniors experiencing persistent pain may develop symptoms of depression, anxiety, or frustration.

Implementing effective pain management strategies contributes to improved emotional health and overall well-being.

5. Sleep Quality and Mental Health

Adequate sleep is essential for mental wellness. Seniors experiencing sleep disturbances or insomnia are at a higher risk of developing mental health issues. Addressing sleep problems positively impacts mood, cognitive function, and emotional stability.

6. Physical Health and Social Engagement

Physical health influences seniors' ability to engage socially. Good physical health allows for active participation in social activities, promoting connections with others and reducing feelings of isolation, thereby benefiting mental health.

7. Chronic Illnesses and Mental Well-being

Managing chronic illnesses is vital for mental wellness. Seniors dealing with long-term health conditions often face emotional challenges. Effective management and treatment of these illnesses play a critical role in preserving mental health.

8.Cognitive Health and Emotional Stability
Maintaining cognitive health is imperative for emotional stability. Seniors experiencing cognitive decline may also exhibit changes in mood or emotional regulation. Strategies that support cognitive function positively impact mental well-being.

Addressing physical health concerns among seniors is crucial for preserving their mental wellness. Encouraging healthy lifestyle choices, promoting regular exercise, ensuring proper nutrition, managing chronic illnesses effectively, and prioritising good sleep hygiene contribute significantly to maintaining both physical and mental health in this demographic.

Exploring the mind-body connection

The mind-body connection refers to the intricate relationship between mental and physical health, showcasing how thoughts, emotions, and physiological states influence each other. Understanding and exploring this connection is essential, especially for seniors over 50, as it significantly impacts their overall well-being.

1. Stress Response and Physical Health

Psychological stress triggers physical responses in the body. Chronic stress can lead to increased cortisol levels, impacting the immune system, cardiovascular health, and even digestion. Understanding stress management techniques aids in mitigating its physical repercussions.

2. Emotions and Physical Health

Emotions have a tangible impact on physical health. Negative emotions like anxiety, sadness, or anger can manifest as physical symptoms, such as headaches, digestive issues, or muscle tension. Cultivating emotional awareness and regulation positively impacts physical health.

3. Pain Perception and Psychological States

Psychological states influence pain perception. Emotions like fear, stress, or depression can exacerbate pain sensations, while positive emotions or relaxation techniques can alleviate discomfort. Managing emotional well-being contributes to better pain management.

4. Placebo Effect and Mind-Body Connection

The placebo effect demonstrates the power of the mind in healing the body. Believing in a treatment's efficacy can lead to actual physical improvements, highlighting the role of mindset in health outcomes.

5. Mental Health and Physical Health Interplay

Mental health conditions like depression or anxiety often have physical manifestations. Depression might lead to fatigue, changes in appetite, or sleep disturbances, while anxiety might cause palpitations or gastrointestinal issues. Treating mental health conditions positively impacts physical health.

6.Mindfulness and its Impact

Practices like mindfulness or meditation emphasise the mind-body connection. These techniques enable individuals to focus on the present moment, calming the mind and subsequently impacting physiological responses like reduced heart rate, lowered blood pressure, and decreased stress levels.

7.Positive Thinking and Health Outcomes

Positive thinking and optimism have shown correlations with improved physical health. Seniors who maintain positive attitudes often experience better cardiovascular health, improved immune function, and a reduced risk of chronic illnesses.

Strategies for promoting physical wellness

Promoting physical wellness among seniors over 50 involves a multifaceted approach encompassing various strategies tailored to their needs and abilities.

1. Regular Exercise Routine
Encouraging seniors to engage in regular physical activity is vital. Activities such as walking, swimming, yoga, or tai chi improve cardiovascular health, enhance flexibility, and maintain muscle strength. Customising exercise plans to accommodate individual abilities is essential for sustained engagement.

2. Strength Training and Resistance Exercises
Incorporating strength training exercises using resistance bands or light weights aids in

maintaining muscle mass and bone density. This is crucial for preventing age-related muscle loss and reducing the risk of osteoporosis.

3.Balance and Flexibility Exercises

Implementing exercises that focus on balance and flexibility, such as stretching routines or balance exercises, helps prevent falls and improves mobility. These exercises are particularly beneficial for seniors to maintain independence and prevent injuries.

4.Healthy Nutrition and Hydration

Encouraging a balanced and nutritious diet is paramount for physical wellness. Seniors benefit from a diet rich in fruits, vegetables, whole grains, lean proteins, and adequate hydration. Proper nutrition supports overall health and vitality.

5.Regular Health Check-ups and Screenings

Stressing the importance of regular health check-ups, screenings, and preventive care is crucial. Monitoring blood pressure, cholesterol levels, and receiving age-appropriate screenings helps in early detection and management of health issues.

6. Good Sleep Hygiene

Educating seniors on the significance of quality sleep is essential. Encouraging consistent sleep schedules, creating a comfortable sleep environment, and practising good sleep hygiene contributes to overall physical health and mental well-being.

7. Managing Chronic Conditions

Effectively managing chronic conditions like diabetes, heart disease, or arthritis is vital. Following prescribed treatments, adhering to medication regimens, and implementing lifestyle modifications help in controlling these conditions and improving quality of life.

8. Stress Reduction Techniques

Teaching stress reduction techniques, such as meditation, deep breathing exercises, or mindfulness practices, aids in managing stress levels.Better physical health overall is correlated with reduced stress.

9.Social Engagement and Physical Activity
Encouraging seniors to engage in social activities that involve physical movement, such as dancing, group fitness classes, or community walks, not only promotes physical wellness but also fosters social connections.

10.Adapting to Age-Related Changes
Assisting seniors in adapting to age-related changes, such as changes in mobility or energy levels, by modifying exercise routines or activities ensures continued participation in physical wellness practices.

11.Promoting physical wellness among seniors

Involves a holistic approach that encompasses exercise, nutrition, preventive care, and stress management. Encouraging these strategies supports their overall health, independence, and vitality as they age.

12. Healthy Lifestyle Choices and Well-being
Lifestyle choices significantly affect the mind-body connection. Regular exercise, a balanced diet, sufficient sleep, and stress management techniques contribute to improved mental and physical health, emphasising the importance of holistic well-being.

Exploring the mind-body connection involves adopting a holistic approach to health care. Integrating strategies that consider both mental and physical aspects of health enables seniors to maintain a balanced and healthy lifestyle, promoting overall well-being in their later years.

CHAPTER 5

Overcoming Stigma and Seeking Support

Overcoming stigma surrounding mental health and seeking support is crucial for seniors over 50 to effectively manage their emotional well-being. Addressing mental health concerns requires understanding, openness, and a shift in societal perceptions. Encouraging individuals to seek support involves various strategies tailored to combat stigma.

1. Education and Awareness

Initiating educational campaigns to debunk myths and misconceptions about mental health among seniors is vital. Providing accurate information through workshops, seminars, or informational materials reduces stigma and fosters a supportive environment.

2. Open Dialogue and Normalization

Encouraging open conversations about mental health within families and communities normalises seeking help. Sharing personal stories or testimonials reduces stigma by showcasing that seeking support is a common and acceptable practice.

3. Promotion of Self-Care Practices

Emphasising self-care practices as a means of maintaining mental health reduces the stigma associated with seeking support. Encouraging activities like meditation, relaxation techniques, or engaging in hobbies promotes mental well-being without attaching negative connotations.

4. Access to Resources and Support Groups

Facilitating access to mental health resources and support groups tailored for seniors creates safe spaces for seeking help. Providing information about helplines, counselling services, or peer support groups fosters a sense of community and reduces feelings of isolation.

5. Collaboration with Healthcare Providers

Collaborating with healthcare providers to prioritise mental health screenings during routine check-ups promotes early identification of issues. Integrating mental health assessments into primary care settings reduces stigma and encourages proactive care.

6. Promotion of Confidentiality and Privacy

Ensuring confidentiality and privacy in seeking support services encourages individuals to feel secure in sharing their concerns. Creating a safe environment where personal information is protected reduces fear of judgement or discrimination.

7. Empowerment through Information

Providing seniors with information about the efficacy of mental health treatments, therapies, and available interventions empowers them to make informed decisions. Knowing that effective help is available encourages seeking support.

8.Cultural Sensitivity and Diversity

Recognizing and respecting diverse cultural beliefs and practices surrounding mental health is crucial. Providing culturally sensitive resources and support acknowledges individual differences and encourages seeking help within culturally appropriate frameworks.

9.Role of Supportive Relationships

Highlighting the role of supportive relationships in mental health encourages seeking support. Emphasising the positive impact of familial, social, or community connections on mental well-being reduces the stigma associated with seeking help.

10.Celebrating Recovery Stories

Sharing success stories of individuals who sought help and successfully managed mental health challenges reduces stigma. Highlighting stories of resilience and recovery instils hope and encourages others to seek support.

Overcoming stigma and encouraging seniors to seek support for mental health requires a concerted effort to foster understanding, provide resources, and create supportive environments. Normalising seeking help empowers individuals to prioritise their mental well-being without fear of judgement or discrimination.

Addressing misconceptions about mental health

Addressing misconceptions about mental health among seniors over 50 is crucial in fostering a more supportive and understanding environment. Dispelling myths and promoting accurate information helps reduce stigma and encourages individuals to seek appropriate support. Here are strategies to tackle these misconceptions:

1. Education and Awareness Campaigns
Implementing educational programs that debunk common myths about mental health is essential. Utilising various mediums such as workshops, seminars, or informative pamphlets helps disseminate accurate information.

2. Open Discussions and Community Forums
Creating safe spaces for open discussions within communities allows for dialogue about mental health. Hosting forums where individuals can share experiences and ask questions fosters understanding and diminishes misconceptions.

3. Sharing Stories and Testimonials
Encouraging individuals who have experienced mental health challenges to share their stories reduces stigma. Personal narratives illustrate that

mental health issues are common and can affect anyone, regardless of age, background, or status.

4. Highlighting the Biological Basis of Mental Health

Emphasising the biological basis of mental health conditions helps combat misconceptions that they're solely due to personal weakness or character flaws. Explaining the role of brain chemistry and genetics in mental health conditions promotes understanding.

5. Promotion of Professional Expertise

Highlighting the expertise of mental health professionals and their ability to provide effective treatments counters misconceptions about the efficacy of seeking help. Promoting the success of therapy, medication, and other interventions demonstrates their value in managing mental health.

6. Addressing Stigma within Cultural Contexts

Acknowledging cultural beliefs and perspectives regarding mental health is crucial. Tailoring education and awareness campaigns to respect diverse cultural viewpoints helps bridge understanding and reduces stigma.

7. Fostering Empathy and Compassion

Encouraging empathy towards individuals facing mental health challenges cultivates a more compassionate attitude. Understanding the difficulties individuals encounter encourages support rather than judgement.

8. Media Representation and Messaging

Working with media outlets to portray mental health issues accurately in movies, TV shows, and news reports is impactful. Responsible portrayal in media helps challenge stereotypes and dispel misconceptions.

9. Integrating Mental Health Education in Schools and Community Centers

Incorporating mental health education into school curriculums and community centre programs normalises conversations and addresses misconceptions from an early age.

10. Providing Accurate Information through Healthcare Providers

Encouraging healthcare providers to discuss mental health during routine check-ups and providing accurate information further educates individuals and reduces misunderstandings.

Addressing misconceptions requires a concerted effort involving education, open dialogue, and cultural sensitivity. By fostering understanding and promoting accurate information, society can create a more supportive environment for individuals dealing with mental health challenges.

Encouraging seeking professional help

Encouraging seniors over 50 to seek professional help for mental health concerns is crucial for their overall well-being. Overcoming barriers and promoting the benefits of professional support involves various strategies:

1.Normalising Seeking Help
Normalising the idea of seeking professional help for mental health issues reduces stigma. Emphasising that seeking help is a proactive step towards better mental health encourages individuals to consider it as a standard part of self-care.

2.Educating on the Benefits of Therapy
Educating seniors on the benefits of therapy or counselling sessions helps in demystifying the process. Explaining how therapy provides a safe

space to express emotions, gain coping strategies, and manage stressors fosters a more positive attitude towards seeking help.

3.Providing Information about Mental Health Professionals

Offering information about mental health professionals such as psychologists, counsellors, or psychiatrists, including their qualifications and areas of expertise, helps in building trust and confidence in seeking professional support.

4.Emphasising Confidentiality and Privacy

Highlighting the confidential nature of therapy sessions reassures individuals about privacy. Knowing that discussions in therapy remain confidential encourages seniors to seek help without fear of judgement or disclosure.

5.Promoting Success Stories

Sharing success stories of individuals who sought professional help and experienced positive outcomes instils hope. Hearing about others' journeys towards improved mental health encourages seniors to consider seeking similar support.

6. Role of Medication and Treatment

Addressing the role of medication and treatment in managing mental health conditions reduces apprehensions. Clarifying that medication, when prescribed by professionals, can complement therapy and aid in symptom management promotes understanding.

7. Facilitating Access to Services

Assisting seniors in navigating the process of finding mental health services and support resources is crucial. Providing information about helplines, support groups, or affordable counselling services facilitates access to help.

8. Encouraging Family and Peer Support

Involving family members or peers who have had positive experiences with mental health professionals encourages seniors to seek similar support. Peer support and encouragement play a pivotal role in breaking down barriers.

9. Highlighting Improved Quality of Life
Emphasising how seeking professional help positively impacts overall quality of life, relationships, and coping strategies encourages individuals to prioritise their mental well-being.

10. Addressing Barriers and Concerns
Addressing specific concerns or misconceptions seniors might have about seeking professional help validates their worries and provides accurate information to alleviate their fears.

Encouraging seniors to seek professional help involves providing accurate information, fostering support networks, and highlighting the benefits of seeking mental health support. By promoting understanding and reducing barriers, individuals can access the necessary resources to improve their mental well-being.

CHAPTER 6

Adapting to Life Changes

Adapting to life changes becomes increasingly important for seniors over 50 as they navigate transitions in various aspects of their lives. Implementing strategies to adapt positively to change involves:

1. Embracing a Growth Mindset
Encouraging a mindset that perceives change as an opportunity for growth and learning fosters resilience. Seniors can view transitions as a chance to explore new experiences and expand their horizons.

2. Maintaining Flexibility and Adaptability
Cultivating flexibility in response to change allows seniors to adjust more readily. Being open to different possibilities and adapting to new

circumstances helps in navigating transitions smoothly.

3. Seeking Support Networks
Engaging with support networks, whether through family, friends, or community groups, provides a sense of belonging during periods of change. These connections offer emotional support and practical guidance.

4. Developing Coping Strategies
Encouraging the development of coping strategies, such as mindfulness, journaling, or relaxation techniques, aids in managing stress associated with life changes. These practices promote emotional well-being.

5. Emphasising Self-Care Practices
Prioritising self-care during transitions is crucial. Encouraging activities like exercise, healthy eating, and adequate rest supports physical and mental well-being, fostering resilience.

6. Setting Realistic Expectations

Encouraging seniors to set realistic expectations during transitions helps manage uncertainties. Recognizing that adjustments take time and allowing oneself space to adapt eases the pressure of change.

7. Maintaining a Sense of Purpose

Emphasising the importance of maintaining a sense of purpose or setting new goals contributes to a positive outlook during transitions. Engaging in meaningful activities fosters a sense of fulfilment.

8. Learning and Skill Development

Encouraging lifelong learning or picking up new skills enhances adaptability. Seniors can explore hobbies, attend classes, or learn new technologies to embrace change more effectively.

9. Acknowledging Emotions and Seeking Help

Validating emotions that arise during transitions and seeking professional help if needed fosters emotional well-being. Accepting and addressing feelings of anxiety, sadness, or uncertainty is crucial for adjustment.

10. Reflecting on Past Resilience
Reflecting on past instances of successfully navigating change reinforces resilience. Seniors can draw upon their past experiences to find strength during new transitions.

Adapting to life changes involves a multifaceted approach that encompasses emotional well-being, social connections, and personal growth. Encouraging a positive attitude towards change empowers seniors to embrace transitions with resilience and optimism.

Managing life transitions and retirement

Managing life transitions, especially retirement, is a significant journey for seniors over 50. Strategies to effectively navigate this period of change involve:

1. Preparation and Planning

Encouraging early planning for retirement allows seniors to envision their post-retirement lifestyle. Financial planning, setting goals, and outlining activities they wish to pursue post-retirement provide a sense of direction.

2. Creating a New Routine

Helping seniors establish a new routine post-retirement fosters a sense of structure and purpose. Encouraging engagement in hobbies, volunteering, or part-time work maintains a sense of fulfilment.

3. Maintaining Social Connections

Emphasising the importance of social connections during retirement is crucial. Encouraging seniors to stay connected with friends, join clubs, or participate in community activities combats feelings of isolation.

4. Financial Management and Budgeting

Supporting seniors in managing their finances and adjusting to potential changes in income post-retirement is essential. Educating them on budgeting and seeking professional financial advice aids in financial stability.

5. Healthcare Planning

Ensuring seniors have healthcare plans in place post-retirement is vital. Assisting in understanding healthcare options, including insurance coverage and Medicare, supports their health needs.

6. Exploring New Opportunities

Encouraging exploration of new opportunities, such as pursuing education, starting a business, or travelling, broadens horizons and adds excitement to the retirement phase.

7. Emotional Preparedness and Self-Care
Addressing the emotional aspect of retirement and the potential psychological impact is crucial. Encouraging self-care practices, stress management techniques, and seeking emotional support promotes well-being.

8. Adjusting to Lifestyle Changes
Assisting in adjusting to changes in lifestyle, such as downsizing, relocation, or changes in daily routines, helps seniors adapt more comfortably to their new circumstances.

9. Exploring Second Career or Part-Time Work
Encouraging seniors to explore second careers or part-time work based on their interests or expertise allows for continued engagement and financial stability.

Navigating life transitions, particularly retirement, involves comprehensive planning and emotional preparedness. Encouraging seniors to embrace this phase as an opportunity for growth, exploration, and new experiences empowers them to transition more smoothly into the next chapter of their lives.

Coping with grief and loss

Coping with grief and loss is a deeply personal experience, especially for seniors over 50 who may face various losses, including the loss of a loved one, health, independence, or a sense of purpose. Strategies to support them during these difficult times involve:

1. Encouraging Expression of Feelings
Creating a safe space for seniors to express their emotions freely without judgement fosters healing. Encouraging them to talk, write, or engage in creative outlets helps in processing emotions.

2. Validating Grief Reactions

Validating diverse grief reactions, including sadness, anger, guilt, or numbness, helps normalise their feelings. Assuring seniors that their reactions are natural aids in coping.

3. Providing Emotional Support

Offering emotional support through active listening, empathy, and companionship helps seniors feel understood and less alone in their grief journey.

4. Maintaining Routines and Structure

Encouraging the maintenance of daily routines provides a sense of stability during an emotionally turbulent time. Structure helps in managing emotions and maintaining a sense of normalcy.

5. Supporting Physical Well-being

Emphasising the importance of physical health through regular exercise, proper nutrition, and adequate rest supports emotional well-being during grief.

6. Encouraging Support Networks
Seniors who are grieving can share their stories and find solace from people who understand them by being connected to family, friends, or support groups.

7. Honouring Memories
Encouraging seniors to honour the memories of their loved ones through rituals, creating memorials, or participating in activities that celebrate the life of the person they've lost fosters healing.

8. Exploring Spiritual or Religious Support
Encouraging seniors to engage in spiritual or religious practices that bring comfort and meaning aids in the grieving process.

9. Allowing Time for Healing

Reminding seniors that grief is a process that takes time and varies for each individual validates their journey. Encouraging patience and self-compassion throughout this process is important.

10. Supporting seniors through grief Involves a compassionate and understanding approach. Acknowledging the uniqueness of each individual's grieving process and providing tailored support enables them to navigate through their loss while finding comfort and healing in their own time.

CHAPTER 7

Creating a Holistic Mental Health Plan

Creating a holistic mental health plan for seniors over 50 involves a comprehensive approach that addresses various aspects of well-being. Here's a breakdown:

1. Physical Activity and Nutrition
Incorporating regular exercise tailored to their abilities improves mood and overall mental health. Coupled with a balanced diet rich in nutrients, it supports brain function and emotional stability.

2. Social Engagement and Support Systems
Encouraging seniors to maintain social connections through family, friends, or community groups

fosters a sense of belonging and reduces feelings of isolation, promoting mental well-being.

3. Mindfulness and Stress Management
Teaching mindfulness techniques like meditation, deep breathing, or yoga helps in managing stress. These practices enhance emotional regulation and reduce anxiety.

4. Cognitive Stimulation and Brain Health
Engaging in activities that challenge the mind, such as puzzles, reading, or learning new skills, supports cognitive health and emotional well-being.

5. Sleep Hygiene and Restorative Sleep
Emphasising the importance of good sleep hygiene ensures adequate rest, which is vital for mental clarity, mood regulation, and overall mental health.

6. Emotional Support and Coping Strategies
Encouraging the development of coping strategies, like journaling, art therapy, or seeking professional

help, provides tools to manage emotions and navigate challenges.

7. Self-Care and Relaxation Techniques
Promoting self-care practices, such as taking breaks, enjoying hobbies, or engaging in nature, rejuvenates the mind and reduces stress.

8. Balancing Work or Activities with Leisure
Supporting a balance between work, leisure, and relaxation prevents burnout and supports mental well-being.

9. Holistic Assessment and Flexibility
Regularly evaluating the effectiveness of the mental health plan and being flexible to adjust strategies based on changing needs ensures it remains effective.

10. Creating a holistic mental health plan
Involves a multi-dimensional approach that addresses physical, social, emotional, and cognitive

aspects of well-being. Encouraging a balance between these elements contributes to a comprehensive and sustainable mental health strategy for seniors.

Building personalised strategies for mental well-being

Building personalised strategies for mental well-being among seniors over 50 involves tailoring approaches to individual needs and preferences. Here's a breakdown:

1. Assessment and Understanding
Begin by understanding the individual's current mental health status, preferences, challenges, and strengths through open conversations or assessments.

2. Identifying Triggers and Stressors

Collaborate to identify specific triggers or stressors that impact mental well-being, such as health concerns, life transitions, or social factors.

3. Setting Realistic Goals

Establish achievable and personalised goals focusing on areas that need improvement or maintenance, such as managing stress, improving sleep, or enhancing social connections.

4. Incorporating Preferred Activities

Integrate activities the individual enjoys into their routine, whether it's physical exercise, creative hobbies, or social engagements, to boost mood and motivation.

5. Encouraging Meaningful Connections

Support maintaining or establishing meaningful relationships that contribute positively to mental health, whether with family, friends, or community groups.

6. Cultivating Mindfulness Practices

Explore mindfulness techniques tailored to the individual's preferences, such as meditation, deep breathing exercises, or guided imagery, to manage stress and anxiety.

7. Developing Coping Strategies

Collaborate on developing coping strategies personalised to handle challenges or emotional distress, which could involve journaling, seeking social support, or engaging in relaxation techniques.

8. Nutrition and Physical Health

Address the importance of a balanced diet and regular physical activity as they significantly impact mental well-being.

9. Regular Evaluation and Adjustment

Continuously assess the effectiveness of strategies and be open to adjusting approaches based on feedback or changes in the individual's circumstances or needs.

Building personalised strategies for mental well-being requires a collaborative and adaptable approach that considers the individual's unique preferences, challenges, and strengths. By tailoring strategies to their specific needs, seniors can develop a comprehensive plan that supports their mental health and enhances their overall well-being.

Resources and tools for ongoing support

Here are various resources and tools tailored to provide ongoing support for the mental well-being of seniors over 50:

1.Support Groups and Community Centers
Local community centres often host support groups, workshops, or social activities tailored for

seniors. They provide opportunities for social interaction and emotional support.

2. Helplines and Hotlines
Mental health helplines and hotlines offer immediate assistance and guidance during emotional crises or when individuals need someone to talk to urgently.

3. Online Mental Health Resources
Websites and online platforms offer mental health information, articles, forums, and virtual support groups catering specifically to seniors.

4. Mobile Applications
Numerous mobile apps focus on meditation, mindfulness, stress reduction, sleep improvement, or cognitive exercises, providing accessible tools for mental wellness.

5. Educational Workshops and Webinars

Organisations frequently organise workshops or webinars covering various mental health topics relevant to seniors, offering educational resources and coping strategies.

6. Therapeutic Services
Accessing therapy or counselling services from licensed professionals, either in-person or via telehealth, provides personalised support for mental health concerns.

7. Community Programs and Activities
Participating in community-based programs, such as art classes, exercise groups, or volunteering opportunities, fosters social connections and promotes mental well-being.

8. Public Libraries and Reading Materials
Libraries often offer books, audiobooks, and resources on mental health, self-help, relaxation techniques, and personal development.

9. Senior Centers and Wellness Programs

Senior centres may organise wellness programs focusing on mental health, including seminars, workshops, and group activities beneficial for mental well-being.

10. Healthcare Providers and Support Services

Engaging with healthcare providers, social workers, or case managers helps in accessing available mental health services and support tailored to individual needs.

These resources and tools serve as ongoing support systems, providing a range of options for seniors to access information, guidance, social interaction, and professional assistance to support their mental well-being on an ongoing basis.

CONCLUSION

"Mental Health for Seniors Over 50" strives to illuminate the path to emotional well-being, offering a comprehensive guide tailored specifically for this vibrant demographic. Throughout these pages, we've explored the intricate landscape of mental health, acknowledging its nuances, challenges, and the transformative power of tailored strategies.

This book serves as a trusted companion, nurturing understanding and empowerment. From unravelling the complexities of mental health in later years to offering insights into navigating life transitions, grief, and fostering a holistic mental health plan, each chapter is a stepping stone towards resilience and vitality.

It's a testament to the significance of personalised strategies, compassionate support networks, and the courage to seek help when needed. Through embracing change, honouring emotions, and celebrating the strengths inherent in every individual, this book endeavours to instil hope and guidance.

As we conclude this journey, may these insights and tools continue to echo as pillars of strength, guiding seniors over 50 towards a life imbued with emotional balance, purpose, and the unwavering belief in the transformative power of prioritising mental well-being. Remember, each step towards mental health is a testament to resilience and a declaration of the innate strength within.

May the lessons learned within these pages foster a life enriched by understanding, support, and the unwavering pursuit of mental well-being for all seniors over 50.

Made in the USA
Coppell, TX
14 August 2024